The Simple Cookbook

How to Boost your Metabolism, Increase your Metabolic Rate and Lose Weight with Mouthwatering Recipes

By

Rina S. Gritton

Acknowledgment

This book has taken years in the making, gathering of information from experience, observations, and meticulous research all in a bid to tackle man's most significant inconveniences. Throughout this journey, I have the privilege to have some of the world's best people stand by me. Looking back and seeing the result of the fruits of my labor and the potential that it has to change lives, I cannot but thank those that made it happen.

To you all, this is a big hug. Thank you.

Copyright © 2019 Rina S. Gritton

The author retains all rights. No part of this document may be reproduced or transmitted in any form or by any means, electronic or mechanical, including photocopying, recording, or by any information storage and retrieval system without permission in writing from the author. The unauthorized reproduction or distribution of this copyrighted work is illegal.

Disclaimer

The information contained in this material is based on years of several types of research by scientists, dieticians, and other professionals in the health field. Whatever you read within the pages of this book is for purely of informational purposes only and is not to be taken as a guide for diagnosis for any psychological or medical condition, nor to treat, mitigate or prevent any disease. Do not discard the professional advice from qualified health care personnel based on the information you get from this book. This book is not intended to be, and you should decide your health based on relevant discussions with a qualified medical doctor or healthcare professional.

Contents

CHAPTER ONE 7

CHAPTER TWO 40

CHAPTER THREE 53

CHAPTER FOUR 70

CHAPTER FOUR 91

CHAPTER FIVE 105

CHAPTER SIX 116

CHAPTER ONE

You must have had a hard time trying to get your weight in check; either getting rid of some excess body weight or bulking up but you never seem to get it right. You have tried out all the diet fads, but nothing ever seems to work for you. The solution to your problem does not lie in the type of diet that you may have decided to try out, the key to unlocking the door to dealing with your yo-yoing weight lies right there in front of you. Your metabolism is most likely the culprit.

What is Metabolism?

That word metabolism must have been heard right from your science classes in high school and all through college if you had a bias for the sciences. It connotes this picture or an image of breaking down of food in the human body, making use of calories and generally expending energy. You could be quite close to the point, but metabolism has a deeper meaning than this simple idea that most of us have.

Metabolism in its simplest definition is the mechanism through which the human body makes use of nutrients that it takes in through food and undergoes biochemical reactions to generate energy for the most minute functioning of the human cell. How the cells of your body carry out their daily activities is determined by the energy that such cells can manufacture and ultimately consume. Think about your body as a machine with many individual parts all working independently and at the same time in unison for the betterment of the whole being. From your skeletal system to your muscular system, the brain to the gastrointestinal tract can only function properly in the way they have been designed to if they can make use of nutrients supplied to them to produce the type of energy material that will be advantageous to their tasks. This is what metabolism is and not how much energy you make use of day in day out. The metabolic process of your body is how your body system generates and makes use of the packets of energy available to it.

When you begin to see your metabolic system as just been more than the amount of energy you consume, then your metabolism becomes more than only energy consumption. Your metabolism becomes a healthy functioning system that has a direct effect on your general wellbeing from how you enjoy your day, how much rest you get, the quality of your epidermal cells, etc. When the cells are supplied continuously with quality nutrients, they perform at their best at all times, which results in the body been healthy. If this situation is otherwise; however, your metabolism takes a hit and gently grinds to a halt to adjust to the poor and low quality of calories that it is being supplied. Energy will be channeled from different parts of the body to parts that need them the more to keep every organ functioning, or a semblance of that. For example, the energy needs of the skin and hair may be forgone and transmitted to the brain. This results in poor skin conditions and dry, breaking hair. The million dollar question here now is, are you putting your metabolic system under undue pressure or actually treating it the way that it should? Your everyday routine goes a long way towards ensuring that your metabolism works perfectly. You may assume it is one heck of a mountain to climb, no; I can assure you that it is not. All you need to do is begin to identify those factors that are causing a stressed metabolic system and affect the proper changes. For you to do this, there is the need to have a proper understanding of your metabolic system and how it functions.

Damaging Habits

As we grow older and become more aged, it is only natural that some of our bodily functions begin, and our metabolism is not excluded. That's the biology of the human body, and with the modern lifestyle that we have all embraced, this process has been put on the fast track. The sad thing here is that ignorance comes to play. Just think about any activity that you perform daily, from the time you wake up, the type of breakfast that you have, the stress you undergo at the workplace can all have detrimental or positive effects on your metabolism.

You may take some of your activities as being "healthy" based on the current fad. You exercise maybe just a bit too much, follow the dietary practices that are in vogue and at the same time hardly ever rest due to the targets you have to meet in building your career. This will inevitably lead to a chain reaction culminating in the total breakdown of your metabolic system. Has it crossed your mind that all the supposedly healthy foods and exercise regimes you are putting your body through are responsible for your current situation? What if I told you that the low-fat diet you are on has adverse effects on your body and that a high-fat diet, a reduced exercising period and some changes to your daily regime may bring about the healing to your metabolism that you so desire? You may have become so stuck in your ways that change does not come easy or you have a more flexible personality such that you can flip the switch and move on to a more healthier lifestyle. Getting different results entails you to do things differently. Before you can begin to make changes, there is the need to identify some of the factors responsible for a faulty metabolism.

Stress

When we talk about stress, generally, what comes to mind are feelings attached to our love life, family problems, work, etc. Stress can be those things, and at the same time, it can be triggered by a lot of elements that have nothing to do with the emotional health of the individual. This wrong notion about what stress is also permeated how you, as an individual view how it relates to your health viz your metabolism. Having a basic understanding of what stress is and how it can be detrimental to your health is the first and most vital step you can take towards healing or preventing having a metabolic breakdown.

Stress in its simplest term is a reaction either external or internal that brings about the release of biochemical substances called hormones such as cortisol and adrenaline. When your body undergoes unfavorable conditions which are certainly almost not natural, these hormones are released into the system to counteract that effect.

When a stressful event occurs, your body is unable to identify what type of stress it is currently undergoing; it simply gives a blanket reaction to whatever form of stress is thrown at it. When stress occurs, and the hormones are released, it usually has a beneficial effect at that moment such as increasing the amount of glucose needed to carry out high energy consuming activities at that time or increase your resistance to pain. These events are not supposed to be a regular occurrence but take a look around you now, and can you honestly pick out one person who does not undergo stressful situations consistently every day? This leads to the stress hormones been always present in the body system leading to severe consequences. Cortisol and adrenaline metabolize useful components of your skeletal and muscular systems, and before long, other body organs begin to suffer the same fate. There is also diversion of valuable energy resources form parts of the body that usually does not demand much, e.g., your gastrointestinal system. Having an idea of the several elements that make up stress is pertinent is putting the condition in check. So what are the common types of stress factors that abound all around us today? Here are a few;

Sleep deprivation and rest; this is one of the most common factors that we can all relate with. With the jet style lifestyle, having to achieve more in a limited time, folks have now put sleep and rest on the back burner. Inevitably, stress becomes a partner to anyone who puts the body under such conditions.

Dietary Habits; having tasty and nutritionally balanced meals regularly is the basis of any human body having a sound metabolic condition. When you begin to try out every new diet, cutting out meals because you don't have the time, restricting some classes of food will ultimately bring massive stress to your system. This may seem a bit awkward considering that dieting, not eating regularly and cutting out some types of nutrient classes are the in thing nowadays, but the fact is that they are causing serious damage to the body even though a lot of people will resist the fact staring at them in the face. Waking up very early to catch the train without time to have a decent breakfast and then gulping several cups of caffeine-loaded drinks all through the day to keep going. At the end of the day, it is most likely that such a person will make abysmal eating choices because hunger clouds our decision-making process leading to the consumption of poor calorific foods. This happens over and over continuously until it becomes a habit, and the stress builds up all over the body.

Psychological stress; this has to do with the emotional wellbeing of any person. If there is fighting between couples, the office space is always under pressure to deliver, and lack of job satisfaction, loss of a family member or friend can be causes of stress. If you are tired emotionally way too often, stress comes in. Stress happens in our everyday life, that's an accepted fact, but when it becomes part and parcel of your waking up process till you go to bed at night, then it becomes a big problem. If by chance you find yourself in such a situation, then it is time you take stock of your life and identify things that matters most to you while doing away with things that won't matter in the next few days.

Lack of Sunlight; avoiding the life-giving rays of the sun is a recipe for depression, reduced thyroid function, tiredness, and other emotional problems. This is triggered by the hormone melatonin, which is produced when you stay more in the dark and don't come out during the day. Not only do you expose yourself to stress, but your body will not be able to produce vitamin D. It is no wonder that during the winter months, some of these symptoms are quite common.

Other stress causing factors includes and not limited to the following;

Over-exercising

Exposure to allergies

Exposure to toxic substances

Mechanical injuries

Infections, etc.

Taking a look at the above-listed stress factors; do you think you can take a wide berth around all of them? That will be simply impossible. What you can do is to consciously try to cut down on the impact of these stressors and if you cannot avoid particular stress and its effects, cut down on another form of stress that you have identified to generally reduce the cumulative effect of the strain on your body.

Stress Reducing Tips

Cutting out stress in your life becomes much easier when you have been able to identify what stresses you out. At this point in time, it is pertinent need to take a step towards achieving a much better outlook on life by trying as much as you can to reduce the stress factors impacting you daily. You will be stunned at the transformation that your health and body undergoes by those seemly little changes you make to your relationship with stress. How do you get started with dealing with a few of the stress factors? Keep reading.

Take Quality Resting Times

You cannot underestimate the healing powers of rest, sleep to be specific on your health. This is a fact that cannot be disputed and has been researched and found to be true. At a minimum, you should have six hours of sleep every day to put all those stress hormones in check and generally make you ready to face a new day without being lethargic. You don't need to rest during the night; there are times during the day that you need to unwind and cut out all activities. This might be a little inconvenient and disturbing for some people, but getting your Rolodex arranged to fit in a little you time which might be 1 hour during the day or 1 day off during the week generally boosts your metabolism and makes your well rested.

Most importantly, ensure that you take your leave period from work as at when due. Do not all because of the monetary inducements to work overtime or fill in for colleagues that have taken their vacation times to sit back at work rather than enjoying yourself, soaking up some sun on the beach and sipping something nice. Take that vacation!

Exercise Reasonably

Engaging in activities is advised as it helps the metabolism of nutrients in the body. The catch here is not to go overboard with the process. This can lead to stressing of the body. There are a lot of health benefits in light exercises that improve your mood, strengthens your heart and other organs in the body. Such activities can be carried out daily and do not stress you out. They include swimming, taking walks in the morning or the evening, and engaging in some yoga.

Avoid Emotional Stress

Emotional stress can be tough to handle because we have become accustomed to it and see it as a part of our daily lives. Friction in your relationship, your thought patterns, workplace politics, and finances could be the primary forms of emotional stress affecting you. When tackling these forms of stress, one does not need to treat it in a black or white fashion, preferably a little bit of adjustment here and there will go a long way in improving your discomfort. Learning how to handle situations that might seem impossible and not to your advantage is one of life's lessons that everyone needs to adapt. Managing your thought patterns and preventing it from been all gloom and doom simply because you assume you have no control whatsoever over a situation can give your state of health a significant boost. At times when these challenges and thought patterns are overwhelming, and you have no control over it despite all your best efforts, it is best that you get some support.

Avoid Toxic Substances

With the advancement in science and technology, everywhere we turn, there are bound to be some form of toxic substances from the food that we eat, water, air, soil, etc. It is almost impossible not to come in contact with toxins, but you can take steps towards ensuring that your body does not become overworked with a massive load of these substances. Be proactive by consuming only food substances that are grown without chemical input, filter the air in your living space, do not eat over processed foods, make use of products that have as little as possible inorganic substances.

Be Careful of Allergens

For those who have allergic reactions to certain substances, it is best that you identify the sources of such allergies and avoid them as repeated exposure to such allergens can result in a stressful pattern to your body. As you continue to look out for your metabolism and it becomes much stronger, you will observe that the intensity of your reaction to some substances may not be as it was in the past. Over time, your immunity has improved, and you can, in no small extent, handle the impact of these substances. This does not, however, give you the green card to go overwhelming your system again as it will only lead to more stress and eventual decline in your metabolic health.

Develop Healthy Eating Habits

Food is, and eating the right portions and type of quality food is the start of having excellent metabolic health. For good health at all times, it is essential that one must consume natural, wholesome food, eat as at when due, avoid overly processed food filled with additives, do not restrict particular classes of food as every food type has its uses by the body.

Bask in the Sun

Thirty minutes to one hour a day outdoors in the sun walking, sitting, and engaging in some activities is encouraged as a way for dealing with depression, vitamin D deficiency, and metabolic disorder. In winter and low sunlight regions, artificial sources of light may come in handy, but nothing beats the natural sun rays.

Avoid Mechanical Stress Factors

If by chance your body has been exposed to some form of injuries or infection, in addition to taking medications to heal, plenty of rest is also needed. Pain causes stress to the body, so it is always advised that one take time out to test to hasten the healing process.

Other Metabolic Stressors
The Gut Microbiome

The number of bacteria, bugs, and other flora that inhabit the human gut system are mind-boggling. We have established a symbiotic relationship with these organisms, and they offer some services for the nutrients that we provide them through the food that we eat. When we look at this situation closely, most of the biology of the human body, the reactions, energy generation, etc. are carried out by other forms of life other than the human life form. The human body has become so dependent on these life forms to carry out the most basic tasks that once there is an imbalance in the microflora of the gut; the human body system goes into a tailspin; from your emotions, immunity to metabolism. The bacteria and flora inhabiting the human gut system are essential to our health, but they have come against a lot of attack with the rise of science. Beneficial bacteria are now on the decline which gives room for harmful gut bacteria to promote the proliferation of those that cause a disruption of the system and lead to a leaky gut syndrome, emotional troubles, diabetes, cardiac and cancer amongst others. So how did we come to find ourselves in this situation?

The type of food that we now eat has undergone drastic turnaround from the whole organic foods rich in antioxidants, and nutrients to the highly over processed foods packed full of additives, coloring agents, preservatives and coloring agents. Look through any shelf at the supermarket, and it is filled with cheap genetically modified food and less of organic foods which are unexplainably more expensive. The harm brought to the gut can only be imagined and not to be experienced. Right from the time that a baby is born, he should be introduced to the "normal" environment to ensure the proper development and management of the gut microbes and by extension the immunity. But this is sadly the case as we now live in a "sterile" world filled with antiseptics, antibacterial, etc. that prevents the child from coming in contact with any type of dirt. A lot of mothers also bypass the breastfeeding process and will instead feed put the child on baby formulas. Sadly, the child loses out on the most essential first encountered in immunity-building early on in life.

The more we consume "chemicals" to make our life easier, but by so doing, we kill off the friendly bacteria in our gut. These changes in the population of the microbes in the gastrointestinal system also bring about changes in the constitution of the wall of the stomach leading to leaky gut syndrome and other forms of digestive disorders. The next stage is having inflammation from the toxic materials that have their way into your bloodstream. Some gut bugs have anti-inflammatory properties, and when their numbers get depleted, those that cause problems with insulin resistance, metabolic disorders, and other ailments.

To keep the balance of your gut microbe to your advantage, make sure that you eat fermented foods, fibers, monosaturated fats and whole foods that have not undergone any form of processing,

Sex Hormones

In as much as the type of food, you eat in relation to how active you can lead to serious weight gain. Also, the hormonal imbalances can also be responsible for this unwanted weight gain. The sex hormone; estrogen is a primary culprit when it comes to weight gain. This hormone, when present in more than needed amounts in the human body, can lead to excessive weight gain. The constant intake of refined sugars as we have come to accept to be the norm now brings about higher than normal levels of estrogen in the body. Some other culprits that can bring about higher estrogen levels in the body are antibiotics, toxic substances in the environment, over processed foods, etc. Males are likely to experience symptoms like an abnormal loss of hairs, bloated or spare tire belly, tiredness, build up of fat, osteoporosis, and a low sex drive. Ladies suffer from very painful menstruation, fibroids, excessive large tender breast, etc.

Here's a little secret. Do you know that the human sex hormones are produced from the cholesterol that you consume through your food? So you now see the reason why you should take in healthy amounts of these substances or brace up for a lot of sexual problems. To prevent this condition and in essence your metabolic health, ensure that you eat a reasonable amount of fiber containing meals daily, take plenty of vegetables, little or no alcohol and exercise moderately.

Metabolic Diseases and Nutrition

There is a majorly noticeable rise in the number of metabolic syndrome all around the world with many people at risk of coming down with the ailment. How can one easily diagnose this syndrome? Some factors are pointers to the presence of the, and once a few are identified in an individual, there is the likelihood that sure a person has a metabolic disorder. However, always visit a certified medical practitioner for proper diagnosis and course of treatment. Here are the common methods for determining the syndrome;

High blood pressure (132/87 mmHg) or any other value higher than this.

Blood sugar (fasting) with a value of 102 mg/dL or higher.

Waist measurement higher than 42 inches in men and 37 inches in women.

Low HDL cholesterol values of 42 mg/dL or lower in males and 52 mg/dL or lower in females.

Blood triglycerides (fasting) of 152 mg/dL or higher.

Listed below are some of the common metabolic diseases;

Wilson's disease

Adrenoleukodystrophy

Diabetes type 1

Gaucher disease

Obesity

Lesch-Nyhan Syndrome

Pancreatic cancer

Refsum disease

Maple syrup urine disease

CHAPTER TWO

Dieting

With the craze about all that we eat and new diets popping up here and there every 5 minutes, you must have convinced yourself not once that the latest bandwagon you are jumping on will solve all your health/weight loss issues. It hasn't worked out that way now, or has it? It's a vicious cycle, and there is no way that you can get a spectacular result by engaging in the same practice. You simply have to break that circle and do something different this time around. Improving your metabolism is making a fundamental change in your lifestyle, and you should see it not as a change to a new diet style. It all about tackling your eating and weight gain or loss in a new way. When you try to keep up with new changes in the dieting sphere, you will almost certainly achieve no substantive change to your problems. It is like having your eyes on a thousand and one targets at the same time instead of focusing on just one.

How do you train yourself to be one-minded in this quest to be fit and healthy? You need to become mindful and conscious of your body and discover how your body responds to changes and knowing what it needs at every point in time. Your body does not need to be put through another grueling change that will almost certainly yield no positive result. Why will you always restrict your body from that healthy and nourishing food just because it is the latest fad in town? These constant changes will inevitably pile up unwanted stress on your body. It is all about you been determined to turning a blind eye whatever dieting regimen is in the news and the pressure that you may come under to follow it. The time to begin focusing and aiming to improve your metabolism is now, a delay can be harmful, and you don't have any idea of what the stress you putting yourself through can result into in the next few hours. The harmful side effects that you may have to deal with includes and not limited to a low sexual drive, skin problems, lethargy, gastrointestinal disorders, and a whole lot of other nasty stuff.

There is no short cut to getting your metabolism up and revving again. The more you keep searching for the easy way out, the more you become despondent and depressed as you never lay your hands on that elusive result. If you do by chance come across any diet that seems to work for you, I can tell you that it will not take care of the main problem you are facing, it will only temporarily step down the symptoms while you rejoice in ignorance.

The human body is a connection of highly inter-related individual units that work in synergy to keep the whole running efficiently. These makes the body highly adaptable to changing internal and environmental stimulus to keep it in a well-regulated balance.

When you decide to begin dieting, this delicate relationship is disrupted. For example when you restrict your calorie intake hoping to burn off excess energy storage in the body, you will not get the desired result because the body has been designed in such a way that when there is a reduction in the amount of calories been consumed, it goes into shut down mode drastically reducing the metabolic rate.

The recommended daily calorie intake for females is 2000 – 2100 calories and 2200 – 2300 calories for men and any significant lower o higher calorie intake will result in a stressed metabolism and its associated health risks. There is a morbid stage play been enacted on the world stage if you carefully observe the reaction to food from different parts of the globe. Third world countries are seriously engaged in ways on how to feed their populations with a lot of people currently facing famine and severe malnutrition and starvation while a majority of folks in the developed countries are literally refusing to eat well on purpose! I can bet you imagine the consequences of such actions on the health of a large percentage of the population.

Health professionals and companies are always in our face, pushing information that underlines their agenda; profits. Eat less and exercise more, take magic pills, cut out these food items, feed more on that. Generally, such advise hurts those who take them. An individual might be healthy and decides to take it a step further to maintain that state of health by practicing some form of dieting. Fast forward to a few months later and said the person is already battling one or more types of debilitating body malfunctioning.

Dieting in itself is not natural, and this is the reason why we fight so hard with our innate reasoning to go ahead with it. Thus the reason why large numbers of times that it doesn't always work out. That is a red flag that is a pointer to the ineffectiveness of a lot of dieting forms. You are not obese because you necessarily overeat or underweight because you don't eat, you can't fix your weight problem by regulating the amount of food you eat or don't eat.

You start with a diet plan, and after a few weeks you begin to see results which in itself are ephemeral, and then you notice a sharp decline in your relative health status. Sticking to a diet plan can be one of the hardest things ever for anyone to go on with for an extended period. This cannot always be attributed to that human nature of getting tired with the monotonous program, but it goes deeper than that. Your body is totally against the dieting process you are putting it through that is why you feel that struggle and rebellion from your body. This is what is called a bio-feed mechanism. Whenever your body reacts negatively or fights a diet, you will get a result that will aggravate your current health issues or bring about situations that did not previously exist. The body has been programmed to keep all systems fully functional in times of scarcity of nutrients thus the reason why during a diet, you find it very hard getting rid of the "excess" body weight and when you eventually do, your body gets back at you with a vengeance and some extra weight for you to deal with.

It has been beaten into us that a few extra pounds will be the death of us and yes we have taken it to be the Holy Grail. If you have a few extra pounds on you, then you are to be blamed for it! Eat less and exercise like a first class Olympian! You should stick to the diet plan, go through all the motions to ensure you remain lean. That's all the advice that you get to hear, not minding the toll it will take on your health. Dieting, however, has impacted not just on your body storage fats, it severely disrupts your metabolism. Here are a few side effects of dieting;

There is a break in the natural bonding your body has with food when it is hungry. That moment when you begin to classify food as being good or bad for you, instead of it being an act of providing essential nutrients for the upkeep of the body, then a severe problem is in the offing. This pattern of eating leads one to have a distorted view of the body, emotional eating patterns, eating disorders, and a feeling of being corrupt if one eats the supposedly "wrong" food. The ideal reason you eat will have been destroyed by this eating pattern. A large percentage of the population has turned a deaf ear to the debilitating dangers that dieting has on the health just so that they can achieve that ultimate body weight. This is not living a healthy life as you become obsessed with counting calories and depriving your body of a wide range of essential nutrients.

When dieting, there is an increased chance of experiencing varied weight levels within a relatively short period of times, and this is potentially more harmful than having a few extra pounds on you. When your weight drops and rises constantly, there is an increased chance of you coming down with metabolic disorders.

There is the chance that you will lose essential body tissues and muscles when you diet in addition to the body fat that you aim to get rid of. The basic materials needed by the body organs to work efficiently will be lost during this process. The severity of the associated condition is dependent on the type of dieting practice one is engaged in, but the bottom line remains that is dangerous.

If you are overweight and you don't practice any form of dieting, you are more at an advantage of getting high blood pressure compared to someone who is also overweight and dieting. This points to the fact that extra weight is not that bad when compared to the stress and health challenges that you may get from dieting.

It may seem to be a daunting task in ridding your body of some extra weight. I can tell you that with the right approach and a healthy relationship with your eating patterns, you can achieve healthy weight loss. Do not be tempted into dieting with the mindset of now trying to be healthy once the weighs have dropped off; this is entering into a rat race that most likely will never end. Do not look at the present situations with a short time frame in mind; instead embrace a long term, lifetime approach to your eating habit and your health.

CHAPTER THREE

Recipes Part 1

Veal Burgers and Green Salad

Ingredients

Burger

1 ½ pound ground veal

½ teaspoon black pepper

Two cloves garlic, crushed

Two small green onions, chopped

Three tablespoons extra virgin olive oil

½ teaspoon of sea salt

4 pounds mushrooms, cleaned and chopped

½ teaspoon parsley

Salad

Two tablespoons apple cider vinegar

1 cup lettuce, chopped

1 cup kale, chopped

One avocado, peeled and pitted

Three tablespoons extra virgin olive oil

One small eggplant, peeled and thinly sliced

Two tablespoon Dijon mustard

½ teaspoon cayenne pepper

½ teaspoon of sea salt

Directions

- Put some extra virgin olive oil into a large saucepan over medium heat.
- Add the chopped onions, mushrooms and garlic.
- Sautee for 2 minutes then add the garlic, spices, and salt. Stir continuously for 5 – 7 minutes.
- Take off the heat and allow cooling.
- Put the mayonnaise, pepper, and spices in a bowl. Mix well.

- Add the eggplant, kale, lettuce, avocado, and olive oil. Toss well and let it stand for 20 minutes.
- Add the mushroom mixture and the veal very well with your hand.
- Form patties to your desired size.
- Place the patties on a prepared grill over medium heat.
- Cook the burgers on each side for 8 – 10 minutes on each side.
- Place the grilled burgers on whole wheat bun cut in half with some of the salad to top.
- Enjoy!

Spicy Scrambled Eggs and Shallots

Ingredients

2 cups shallots, thinly sliced

½ teaspoon jalapeno

Two cloves garlic, minced

½ teaspoon ginger, freshly grated

Six egg whites

Two tablespoons extra virgin olive oil

½ teaspoon lemon juice

½ teaspoon of sea salt

½ teaspoon thyme

½ teaspoon curry

One small carrot, grated

Directions

- Add some olive oil to a large saucepan. Sauté the shallots and garlic for about three minutes.
- Add the peppers, carrots and other spices and stir well. Cook for about one minute.
- Pour in the egg whites, stir and cook for about one minute.
- Pour the egg onto a place and drizzle some of the lemon juice over it.

- Sprinkle some fresh basil and parsley.
- Serve warm and enjoy!

Tamil Noodles

Ingredients

4 cups wild rice

Two green onions, thinly sliced

½ teaspoon thyme

½ teaspoon curry

Two tablespoons extra virgin olive oil

½ teaspoon oregano

4 pounds boneless chicken breasts, sliced

2 cups Brussels sprouts

3 cups vegetable broth

One carrot, thinly sliced

1 cup kale, thinly sliced

Sea salt

Sauce

1 ½ cup vegetable broth

One tablespoon ginger, freshly grated

Two cloves garlic, minced

One teaspoon paprika

½ teaspoon chili

Directions

- Cook the wild rice following the instructions on the pack.
- Add all the ingredients for the sauce in a bowl, combine well and keep.
- Add the olive oil to a large pan over medium heat. Introduce the chicken and stir fry for about 6 – 8 minutes. Take out the chicken and allow to cool.
- Add the onions, sprouts, spices and some broth to the pan. Cook for about 4 – 6 minutes while stirring continuously.
- Add the vegetables and cook for another 1 minute.

- Pour in the sauce into the pan with the vegetables, rice, and chicken.
- Cook on low heat for another 3 minutes.
- Serve warm and enjoy!

Walnut Crusted Salmon with Zucchini

Ingredients

½ cup whole wheat bread crumbs

One teaspoon black pepper

½ cup chopped walnut

One tablespoon basil

1 ½ teaspoon dill

½ cup extra virgin olive oil

12 salmon fillets, boneless, skin-on

2 cups zucchini, thinly sliced

½ teaspoon oregano

½ teaspoon paprika

Sea salt

Directions

- Preheat oven to 385 degrees.
- Add the walnuts, some dill, basil, bread crumbs, sea salt and spices to a bowl. Combine well then add some olive oil and mix well again.
- Apply some olive oil to a baking sheet and place the salmon fillets on it. Sprinkle some pepper and salt over the fish.
- Sprinkle the walnut mixture over the fish and gently apply some pressure to it so that the walnut mixture sticks to the fish.
- In another bowl, add the zucchini with some pepper, salt, and olive oil. Toss to combine well.
- Arrange the zucchini around the fish.
- Bake for 7 – 10 minutes.

- Serve warm.

Grilled Turkey Sausages with Green Onions

Ingredients

2 cups shallots, thinly sliced

One large white onion, thinly sliced

One large yellow bell pepper, quartered, seeds removed

16 3-ounce cooked turkey sausages

8 cups basmati rice, cooked

½ teaspoon black pepper

Three cloves garlic, minced

½ teaspoon ginger, grated

One teaspoon fresh parsley

½ teaspoon curry

One teaspoon lemon juice

Sea salt

Directions

- Grill onions, shallots and bell pepper over medium heat for 10 – 12 minutes. Turn intermittently.
- Mix the lemon juice, pepper and other species in a bowl.
- Introduce the vegetables to the lemon juice mixture and parsley. Toss properly.
- Grill the turkey sausages for about 13 – 15 minutes. Turn the sausages regularly until well cooked.
- Cut the sausages and move to a flat, large plate.
- Serve with the basmati rice with the grilled shallots, onions and peppers.
- Enjoy!

Spicy Egg Benedict

Ingredients

Egg Benedict

Six slices cooked bacon

Six poached organic eggs

Two toasted whole wheat muffins halved

3 cups spinach, lightly steamed

Hollandaise Sauce

¼ teaspoon paprika

1/8 teaspoon oregano

One clove garlic, minced

1 ½ tablespoon lemon juice

Four tablespoons extra virgin olive oil, warm

Four large organic egg yolks

½ teaspoon jalapeno

Sea salt

Directions

Hollandaise Sauce

- Add the egg yolks, spices and lemon juice to a high powered food processor.
- Blend at low speed for about one minute.
- Gently pour in the warm olive oil and blend on low speed for 30 seconds.

Egg Benedict
- Arrange the individual parts, apply some of the hollandaise sauce over it.
- Serve and enjoy!

Venetian Tuna Salad

Ingredients

12-ounces tuna, drained

½ cup white onion, chopped

Three tablespoons extra virgin olive oil

½ cup green olives pitted

One tablespoon parsley

3 cups spinach, chopped and steamed

Two tablespoons lemon juice

½ teaspoon cayenne pepper

One clove garlic, crushed

One small eggplant, thinly sliced

Sea salt

Directions

- Add the tuna, eggplants, olives, garlic, and onions to a bowl. Combine thoroughly.
- Introduce the lemon, parsley and olive oil to the bowl.
- Add the spices.
- Combine well.
- Serve with steamed spinach.

Kale Salad with Grilled Pork Sausages

Ingredients

18 3 – ounces pork sausages

5 cups kale, chopped

Four tablespoons lemon juice

2 cups spinach, chopped

½ cup fresh parsley, chopped

½ cup fresh basil, chopped

½ teaspoon black pepper

½ teaspoon yellow pepper

One red bell pepper, sliced

Three cloves garlic, minced

One large white onion, thinly sliced

½ teaspoon oregano

One tablespoon extra virgin olive oil

¼ teaspoon curry

¼ teaspoon turmeric powder

Sea salt

Directions

- Place the sausages in a large bowl and sprinkle with pepper, salt, turmeric, and curry.
- Allow sitting for 10 minutes.

- Grill the sausage for 7 – 10 minutes over medium heat while turning regularly.
- Remove the sausage from the grill and place on a flat plate.
- Add the kale, spinach, spices, lemon juice, olive oil, and toss well.
- Slice the sausage and serve with the kale salad.
- Serve and enjoy!

Black-eyed beans, Spinach and Chia Cakes

Ingredients

2 cups kale, chopped

3 cups spinach, chopped

2 cups black-eyed peas, cooked

Five cloves, garlic, minced

4 cups cooked chia

Six egg whites

One teaspoon curry

½ teaspoon cayenne pepper

½ teaspoon oregano

½ teaspoon paprika

½ teaspoon coriander

Four tablespoons lemon juice, freshly squeezed

Sea salt

Directions

- Preheat oven to 385 degrees.
- Pour the cooked peas into a high powered food processor and blitz until creamy smooth.
- Put the kale and spinach into a bowl. Pour in the cooked peas into the bowl with the vegetables.
- Add in the spices, salt, chia, and egg whites. Combine thoroughly.

- Apply some baking spray on a baking sheet.
- Form patties from the chia mixture and place it on the baking sheet.
- Bake for 18 – 22 minutes while turning regularly.
- Serve warm with a drizzle of lemon juice.

CHAPTER FOUR

Recipes Part 2

Cod with Veggies

Ingredients

3 (6-ounce) cod fillets

One teaspoon black pepper

½ teaspoon cumin

½ teaspoon coriander

Two cloves garlic, minced

1 cup eggplant, thinly sliced

1 cup yellow corn, frozen

1 cup carrots, thinly sliced

1 cup kale, chopped

½ cup basil

One small white onion, sliced

One tablespoon extra virgin olive oil

Five tablespoons lemon juice, freshly squeezed

½ teaspoon oregano

Sea salt

Directions

- Add the pepper, coriander, garlic some salt and cumin in a bowl. Combine well.
- Apply some of the mixtures on the fish.
- Apply the olive oil to a large saucepan and cook the fish over medium heat, 3 – 5 minutes on each side.
- Pour the vegetable ingredients into a bowl and pour in the spice mixture. Toss and combine well.
- Serve the salad with the fish.
- Enjoy!

Garlic Poached Salmon with cole slaw

Ingredients

Quinoa

2 cups quinoa

4 cups boiling water

Garlic Paste

Six cloves garlic, minced

Two teaspoons curry powder

One teaspoon turmeric

½ teaspoon black pepper

½ teaspoon cayenne

½ cup basil, chopped

One teaspoon ginger, grated

One large green onion, chopped

½ teaspoon paprika

Salmon and Slaw

2 cups Brussels sprouts

Six 6-ounce salmon filets

Two cloves garlic, minced

2 cups vegetable broth

1 cup eggplant, thinly sliced

One tablespoon balsamic vinegar

One large yellow bell pepper, thinly sliced

Sea salt

Directions

- Preheat oven to 300 degrees
- Pour the quinoa, salt, and water into a baking dish. Seal the pan with a baking foil.
- Put the onions, garlic and ginger, in a foil and wrap it.
- Place the baking dish with the rice and the foil with the onion into the oven.
- Bake for 70 minutes.
- Add the roasted onion mixture to a food processor and the other garlic paste ingredients. Blend at high speed until a fine paste is formed.

- Add the broth to a large saucepan, four tablespoons of the garlic paste and spices. Add the salmon and cook on low heat for 10 – 12 minutes.
- Place all the ingredients for the slaw into a bowl and combine well.
- Place one fillet each into a bowl, add some of the fish liquid to it. Ladle some of the slaws onto the fish liquid mixture.
- Serve with the cooked quinoa and enjoy!

Fat Burning Sushi Bowl

Ingredients

3 cups brown rice

Three 6-ounce halibut filet

Three tablespoons grapeseed oil

One teaspoon cayenne pepper

One teaspoon tamari

½ tablespoon tahini

One teaspoon balsamic vinegar

Two cloves garlic, minced

One nori sheet, crushed

One teaspoon ginger, grated

2 cups shallots, chopped

1 cup eggplant, thinly sliced

One teaspoon sesame oil

One teaspoon sesame seeds

3 drops stevia

One teaspoon black pepper

Directions

- Cook the rice following instructions on the pack.
- Put the rice in the fridge to cool.
- Prepare the sauce by adding vinegar, sesame oil, garlic, tamari, ginger, pepper, tahini, and stevia in a bowl.

- Pour the grapeseed oil into a large pan and heat. Gently place the spiced halibut fillet into the oil and cook each side for about 2 minutes each. Remove it from the oil and allow to cool.
- Place some of the halibut, eggplant, rice, shallots, nori, etc. into a bowl.
- Apply the dressing ingredients and enjoy!

Green Vegetables with Beef

Ingredients

2 pounds smoked beef

Two packs of frozen mixed vegetable ingredients

½ teaspoon oregano

½ teaspoon paprika

One tablespoon extra virgin olive oil

Sea salt

Directions

- Cut the meat into four equal parts and place into a large pot. Add 2 cups of water and cook on medium heat for about 30 minutes.
- Pour in the vegetables, spices, and salt.
- Cook for 10 minutes.
- Serve warm and enjoy!

Irish Potatoes Chips

Ingredients

Four large Irish Potatoes

½ teaspoon garlic powder

½ teaspoon jalapeno pepper

½ teaspoon of sea salt

Directions

- Preheat oven to 300 degrees.
- Peel the potatoes, wash and thinly slice the potatoes.

- Put the potatoes and the spices into a large bowl.
- Toss well to combine all the ingredients.
- Place the chips on a baking foil.
- Bake for 35 – 45 minutes or until crispy.
- Enjoy!

Shangai Chops

Ingredients

Eight boneless pork chops

Three tablespoons extra virgin olive oil

One teaspoon garlic powder

1½ tablespoons lemon juice, freshly squeezed

A ½ cup of coconut milk

1/ 2 teaspoon ginger powder

½ teaspoon soy sauce

One tablespoon honey

Directions

- To a bowl, add the honey, soy sauce, ginger powder, coconut milk lemon juice, and olive oil.
- Place the pork chops into a Ziploc bag and pour in half of the marinade into it.
- Place the bag in the fridge overnight or allow to sit for 8 – 10 hours.
- Grill the chops on high heat, 10 – 15 minutes on each side while applying some of the remaining marinades to the chops.
- Serve immediately with a side of salad.
- Enjoy.

Grilled Tuna Fillet

Ingredients

Four large tuna fillets with skin on

Three cloves garlic, crushed

Two tablespoons balsamic vinegar

½ lemon, freshly squeezed

One teaspoon black pepper

½ teaspoon thyme

½ teaspoon coriander

½ teaspoon smoked paprika

Sea salt

Directions

- Using a brush, generously apply the vinegar to the tuna.
- Combine the spices and other ingredients in a bowl.
- Sprinkle the spice mixture to the tuna.
- Grill the fish fillet for about 10 -12 minutes on each side.
- Remove tuna from heat and serve warm with your choice of side dish.

Prawn and Kale Salad

Ingredients

Four tablespoon Dijon mustard

1 pound prawn, cleaned, deveined and cooked

½ cup black olives pitted and halved

2 cups kale, chopped

Two tablespoons lemon juice

½ cup cilantro, chopped

One teaspoon black pepper

2 cups Brussels sprouts

Two cod fillets, chopped

One small green onion, thinly sliced

Sea salt

Directions

- Heat some water and salt in a large saucepan and pour in the sprouts. Cook for 2 minutes and then sieve

- and run the sprouts through cold water.
- Add the cod, olives, mustard, lemon juice and spices to a food processor. Blend at high speed until creamy smooth.
- Put the prawn, kale and other veggies into a bowl. Add the fish dressing.
- Toss well and serve.
- Enjoy!

Fried Spicy Crawfish

Ingredients

2 pounds crawfish, cleaned

½ teaspoon ginger powder

¼ teaspoon oregano

½ teaspoon jalapeno

½ teaspoon cumin

½ teaspoon garlic powder

Three eggs, lightly whisked

1 cup extra virgin olive oil

Sea salt

Directions

- Combine all the necessary spices in a large bowl.
- Place a large saucepan over medium heat and pour in the olive oil.
- Pour some of the whisked eggs over the crawfish and gently mix thoroughly with your hands.
- Pour in the mixed spices and mix well to coat thoroughly.
- Pour in the crawfish into the oil and fry for 3 – 5 minutes or until your desired taste is achieved.
- Serve warm with some greens.
- Enjoy!

Zucchini Green Omelet

Ingredients

2 cups green peas

1 cup kale, chopped

Four egg whites, lightly whisked

One large green onion, chopped

One tablespoon extra virgin olive oil

One small carrot, grated

½ teaspoon cayenne pepper

½ teaspoon garlic powder

½ cup broccoli florets

Sea salt

Directions

- Sauté the vegetables and spices in olive oil over medium heat for about 2 minutes. Remove the vegetables and set aside.
- Whisk the eggs into the pan over medium heat. Cook for about 90 seconds.

- Gentle arrange back the sautéed vegetables back onto the egg and gently cover it with one side of the egg.
- Remove from the pan and serve warm.

Chocolate French Toast

Ingredients

Two slices whole wheat bread

½ teaspoon cumin

½ teaspoon chocolate powder

Two egg whites

One teaspoon lemon juice

¼ teaspoon black pepper

One tablespoon honey

¼ cup mixed berries

One tablespoon extra virgin olive oil

Sea salt

Directions

- Combine the egg white and spices in a bowl.
- Dip the bread in the egg mixture for about 30 seconds.
- Heat the extra virgin olive oil over medium heat in a large saucepan.
- Place the bread in the pan and cook both sides lightly.
- In another pan, pour in the mixed berries and stir over low heat for about one minute. Pour in the lemon juice and honey.
- Stir well and turn in the mixture over the toasted bread.
- Serve warm and enjoy!

Brussels sprouts and Chia

Ingredients

1 cup chia

One small green onion, chopped

One teaspoon cumin

¼ dill, chopped

1 ½ cup Brussels sprouts

1 cup cilantro

1 cup kale

½ teaspoon cayenne

½ teaspoon black pepper

½ teaspoon ginger, grated

One large tomato, sliced

½ cup eggplant, peeled, seeded and diced

Sea salt

Three cloves garlic, crushed

½ cup lemon juice, freshly squeezed

One medium sized red bell pepper, sliced and deseeded

Directions

- Gently wash the chia and pour it into a pot. Add 2 ½ cups of water and

- some salt. Allow to boil, then let it simmer for 17 to 20 minutes. Take it off the heat and then gently stir it.
- In another pot, cook the sprouts in 2 cups of water and then allow simmer for 10 minutes. Drain and then pour in the sprouts with the chia.
- Combine the mixture thoroughly in a large bowl and refrigerate for 30 minutes.
- Add the other ingredients and spices to the chia-sprouts mixture.
- Combine well using a wooden spatula.
- Garnish with the sliced eggplants and tomatoes.
- Serve and enjoy!

Halibut, Citrus and Lentils Salad

Ingredients

3 pounds halibut fillet, steamed

Two tablespoons orange juice, freshly squeezed

Two tablespoons grape, freshly squeezed

One tablespoon balsamic vinegar

½ cup pineapple, cubed

1 cup spinach

One small white onion

Sea salt

½ teaspoon oregano

½ cup zucchini, peeled and diced

½ cup kale

1 cup lentils

Directions

- Add the halibut, vegetables, and other ingredients to a large salad bowl.
- Pour in the juices and toss well to combine correctly.
- Serve immediately or refrigerate.

- Enjoy!

CHAPTER FOUR

Recipes Part 3

Chicken Tortilla Wrap

Ingredients

1 cup lean ground chicken

½ teaspoon oregano

½ teaspoon black pepper

One clove garlic, minced

One small onion, chopped

¼ teaspoon paprika

One tablespoon extra virgin olive oil

1 cup of mixed vegetables

Sea salt

Directions

- Add the extra virgin olive oil to a large skillet over medium heat and add the chicken and spices.
- Cook for 4 – 6 minutes.

- Spread the tortilla and add the vegetables to it.
- Add the chicken and fold the tortilla.
- Serve and enjoy!

Yam and Beans Soup

Ingredients

One small yam, peeled and diced

2 cups brown beans, drained and rinsed

Three cloves garlic, minced

½ pound chicken gizzard

One teaspoon black pepper

½ teaspoon turmeric

One tablespoon ginger, grated

Three large tomatoes, diced

Six tablespoons vegetable broth

One teaspoon oregano

One large red onion, sliced

½ teaspoon cumin

One teaspoon coriander

One teaspoon basil, dried

3 cups chicken broth

Sea salt

Directions

- Put the yam and gizzard into a pot with the chicken broth
- Cook over medium heat until the yam and gizzard are soft.
- Add the beans and other ingredients.
- Cook for another 15 – 20 minutes.
- Reduce the heat and allow simmering for 5 minutes.
- Add salt to taste.
- Serve warm and enjoy!

Turkey and Quinoa Soup

Ingredients

3 cups vegetable broth

5 cups vegetable broth

3 pounds skinless, boneless turkey breast

½ teaspoon black pepper

1 cup quinoa

Sea salt

1 cup eggplant, cubed

One large green onion, diced

1 cup, eggplant, cubed

2 cups broccoli florets

Three cloves garlic, crushed

½ teaspoon cayenne

1/2teaspoon cumin

½ teaspoon paprika

1 cup cilantro

½ cup basil

Directions

- Add the broths and 3 cups of water to a large pot.
- Add the turkey and other ingredients to the pot.

- Cook on high heat till it begins to boil.
- Turn down the heat and allow to simmer for 40 – 50 minutes.
- Put in the vegetables and quinoa to the pot.
- Increase the heat to medium and cook for another 30 – 40 minutes.
- Serve warm and enjoy!

Beef and Spinach Bowl

Ingredients

6 cups beef broth

1 cup onions, chopped

1 cup arugula, chopped

1 cup broccoli florets

3 cups spinach

1 cup wild rice, cooked

Two cloves garlic, minced

One teaspoon basil

3 pounds smoked beef, cubed

One teaspoon black pepper

½ teaspoon cumin

1/2teaspoon paprika

One tablespoon balsamic vinegar

Sea salt

Directions

- Pour the broth to a large pot and introduce the vegetables, spices, and salt to the pan.
- Allow boiling then reduce the heat to simmer for 10 – 15 minutes.
- All to cool.
- Spice the beef with vinegar, salt, cumin, garlic and pepper in a bowl.
- Pour the beef contents into a large baking pan and bake at 395 degrees for 35 to 40 minutes.

- Serve the rice, vegetable, and beef in a bowl in almost equal portions.
- Serve and enjoy!

Chorizo Sausage with Macaroni

Ingredients

One pack macaroni

1 cup eggplant, cubed

1 cup zucchini, cubed

12 ounces Chorizo sausage

1 cup spinach

One medium sized onion, diced

½ teaspoon coriander

½ teaspoon black pepper

Two cloves garlic, minced

One tablespoon extra virgin olive oil

Sea salt

Directions

- Cook the macaroni by going through the instructions on the pack.

- Cube the sausage and sauté in a large saucepan. Add the onions, garlic, spices and two tablespoons of water.
- Cook for about 2 minutes.
- Add the vegetable mixture and cook for a further 2 minutes.
- Pour in the already cooked macaroni and stir well to combine.
- Serve warm and enjoy!

Duck and Brown Rice

Ingredients

3 cups vegetable broth

2 pounds boneless, skinless duck breast

1 ½ cup brown rice

One small white onion, diced

½ teaspoon paprika

Two cloves garlic, crushed

½ teaspoon oregano

Three large tomatoes

½ teaspoon black pepper

One teaspoon basil

1 cup lentils

1 cup black-eyed peas

Sea salt

Two tablespoons extra virgin olive oil

Directions

- Put the duck first into a slow cooker followed by the rice and other ingredients.
- Cook on low heat setting for 7 – 8 hours.
- Serve warm and enjoy.

Turkey Bacon with Arugula

2 cups arugula, chopped

One teaspoon balsamic vinegar

Six slices turkey bacon

One tablespoon Dijon mustard

½ cup eggplant

Sea salt

One tablespoon extra virgin olive oil

Directions

- Cook the bacon in olive oil over medium heat for 3 minutes on each side.
- Spice up the arugula and eggplant with vinegar, mustard, and salt.
- Serve veggies and turkey bacon immediately.
- Enjoy.

Smoked Chicken Breast and Lettuce Wrap

Ingredients

1 pound smoked, boneless chicken breast

Six large romaine leaves

One teaspoon apple cider vinegar

Two tablespoons Dijon mustard

One teaspoon basil

One teaspoon black pepper

½ teaspoon oregano

Directions

- Apply the mustard on the lettuce leaves.
- Then put the chicken on it.
- Sprinkle the spices and drizzle the vinegar over it.
- Wrap up the lettuce and serve.
- Enjoy!

Tuna Veggie Soup

Ingredients

2 pounds tuna fillet

10 cups of frozen mixed vegetables

One large red onion, chopped

Five cloves garlic, minced

One tablespoon cilantro

½ teaspoon rosemary

10 cups fish broth

½ teaspoon curry

½ teaspoon thyme

One teaspoon basil

½ teaspoon paprika

One teaspoon black pepper

Seas salt

Directions

- Add all the ingredients to a extra large stockpot.
- Allow boiling on high heat for 3 minutes then reduce the heat and let to simmer for 50 – 60 minutes.
- Stir well and serve.
- Enjoy!

Vegetable Soup

Ingredients

10 cups of mixed vegetables

3 pounds veal

5 cups beef broth

5 cups vegetable broth

Two large onions, diced

Three large tomatoes, diced

One teaspoon garlic powder

One teaspoon ginger powder

One teaspoon oregano

½ teaspoon rosemary

½ teaspoon cumin

Sea salt

One tablespoon extra virgin olive oil

Directions

- Pour the extra virgin olive oil into a large non-stick skillet.
- Brown the veal over medium heat for about 3 – 5 minutes on each side.
- Place the veal into a slow cooker and add the other ingredients.
- Seal the pot and cook on low heat setting for 7 – 9 hours.

- Serve warm and enjoy.

CHAPTER FIVE

Recipes Part Four

Peppered Salmon Fillet

Ingredients

8 ounces salmon fillet

1 ½ tablespoon lime juice

½ teaspoon rosemary

½ teaspoon garlic powder

½ teaspoon black pepper

½ teaspoon chili pepper

½ teaspoon basil

Sea salt

Directions

- Preheat oven to 315 degrees
- Combine all your spices and salt in a bowl.
- Gently arrange the fish on a greased baking foil and apply the marinade on it.

- Bake for 25 – 35 minutes.
- Serve warm with a side of salad.

Tuna Fillet with Steamed Arugula

Ingredients

8 ounces tuna fillet

2 cups arugula, chopped

1 ½ tablespoon balsamic vinegar

One teaspoon chili pepper

Sea salt

One teaspoon Dijon mustard

½ teaspoon paprika

½ teaspoon rosemary

Directions

- Preheat broiler.
- Combine spices and salt.
- Apply the marinade over the fish.
- Allow it to sit for 20 – 30 minutes.
- Set the fish into the broiler and cook for 10 – 12 minutes.

- Put in the arugula and steam for a further 3 – 5 minutes.
- Sprinkle some spices and salt over the vegetable.
- Serve warm and enjoy.

Stuffed Green Bell Pepper

Ingredients

2 pounds halibut fillet

Four cloves garlic, minced

Six green bell pepper

One large white onion, chopped

Two tablespoons, cilantro

½ teaspoon rosemary

½ teaspoon cumin

Sea salt

½ teaspoon black pepper

½ teaspoon chili

1 cup kale, chopped

One tablespoon extra virgin olive oil

Directions

- Preheat oven to 350 degrees.
- Add the extra virgin olive oil to the pan and cook the fish over medium heat. Add the spices and the herbs.
- Cook for 3 – 5 minutes.
- Add the kale and cook for another 1 minute.
- Take off the heat and allow to cool.
- Cut away the head of each bell pepper and deseed.
- Stuff the pepper with the fish mixture.
- Place the stuffed bell pepper in a baking dish and add three tablespoons of water to the baking dish.
- Seal the baking dish with a foil.
- Bake for 45 – 55 minutes.

- Remove the foil and heat for another 5 minutes.
- Remove the fish from the oven and allow to cool for about 5 minutes before serving.
- Enjoy!

Smoked Halibut and Asparagus

Ingredients

2 pounds smoked halibut fillet

1 ½ teaspoon lime juice

½ teaspoon dill

2 cups asparagus, chopped

½ teaspoon jalapeno

Sea salt

½ teaspoon oregano

Directions

- Pour the asparagus into a bowl an sprinkle the spices over it. Also, drizzle with the lime juice.

- Arrange the fish and asparagus and serve immediately.

Arugula Hummus Toast

Ingredients

Two slices whole wheat bread

½ cup arugula, thinly sliced

One small onion, thinly sliced

One small red tomato, sliced

One clove garlic, minced

Two tablespoons hummus

¼ teaspoon rosemary

¼ teaspoon white pepper

Sea salt

Directions

- Lightly toast the bread and spread some of the hummus over the bread.
- Put some of the arugulas over the hummus and sprinkle the spices over it.

- Serve.

Prawn Salad

Ingredients

3 ounces cooked prawn

3 cups of mixed vegetables

½ teaspoon basil

½ teaspoon oregano

One medium-sized tomato, sliced

Two tablespoons hummus

One teaspoon apple cider vinegar

½ teaspoon parsley

½ cup yellow corn, cooked

Sea salt

Directions

- Combine all the ingredients into a bowl.
- Toss well.
- Serve immediately or refrigerate.

Brussels sprouts Stew

Ingredients

8 cups Brussels sprouts, cooked

Four cloves garlic, minced

One small onion, chopped

Two tablespoons extra virgin olive oil

One teaspoon black pepper

½ cup yellow corn, cooked

½ cup carrot, grated

1 cup beef broth

One tablespoon tamari

½ teaspoon ginger, grated

Sea salt

Directions

- Sauté the onions and garlic in olive oil over medium heat in a large saucepan for 2 minutes.
- Add the sprouts and other ingredients.

- Let it cook for 3 – 5 minutes.
- Add the broth and allow simmering for a few minutes.
- Serve warm.

Smoked Pork chops with Veggies Stir Fry

Ingredients

1 pound smoked pork chops, cubed

Three tablespoons extra virgin olive oil

8 cups of mixed vegetables

Two teaspoons cilantro

One large onion, chopped

Four cloves garlic, minced

1 cup lentils

1 cup Brussels sprouts

One pack spaghetti

½ teaspoon black pepper

½ teaspoon paprika

One teaspoon ginger, grated

Directions

- Stir fry the onions and garlic in olive oil over medium heat until golden brown.
- Add the vegetables and spices for 2 minutes.
- Add the pork chops and cook for about 5 minutes.
- Prepare the spaghetti according to the instructions on the pack.
- Serve warm with the stir-fried pork chops.

Sautéed Arugula

Ingredients

4 cups arugula, chopped

½ teaspoon chili

¼ teaspoon cumin

Sea salt

Two tablespoons extra virgin olive oil

Directions

- Heat the extra virgin oil over medium heat in a large saucepan.
- Add the arugula and other ingredients and stir fry for abou2 – 4 minutes.
- Serve warm.

CHAPTER SIX

Fat Burning Drinks

Coconut Cilantro Water

Ingredients

4 cups of coconut water

Three tablespoons lemon juice

½ cup cilantro

½ cup mixed berries

Ice cubes

Directions

- Pour all the ingredients into a high powered blender.
- Blend at high speed 1 minute.
- Serve chilled.

Strawberry Flavored Chia Water

Four strawberries

Two tablespoons chia

6 cups cold water

½ teaspoon ginger, grated

Directions

- Add all the ingredients to a jar.
- Seal and shake well.
- Refrigerate for about 20 minutes, then shake again.
- Drink within 12 – 18 hours.

Cucumber Vinegar Water

Ingredients

1 cup cucumber, sliced

Two tablespoons apple cider vinegar

Two mint leaves

One tablespoon ginger, grated

Water

Ice cubes

Directions

- Add the cucumber to a large jar followed by other ingredients.
- Add the ice cubes and water.
- Let it sit for 15 – 20 minutes.

- Drink immediately or refrigerate for a few hours.

Ginger Tea Smoothie

Ingredients

Two tablespoon ginger, grated

One clove garlic, minced

Two tablespoons honey

Two tablespoons lemon juice

Three tablespoons Greek yogurt

¼ teaspoon black pepper

1 cup extra strong green tea

Ice cubes

Directions

- Add all the ingredients to a high powered blender.
- Blend for 1 minute.
- Serve chilled.

Rejuvenating Drink

Ingredients

1 cup pineapple, cubed

One apple, cored and sliced

½ eggplant, sliced

½ cucumber, sliced

1 cup of water

½ teaspoon ginger, grated

½ teaspoon turmeric

½ cup kale

One teaspoon apple cider vinegar

Ice cubes

Directions

- Pour all your ingredients into a food processor.
- Blend until smooth.
- Serve chilled.

Fat Blaster

Ingredients

One tablespoon ginger, grated

Three large apples

½ teaspoon turmeric

½ cup kale

½ cup arugula

One mint leaf

Two tablespoons fat-free yogurt

1 cup of water

Ice cubes

Directions

- Add all the ingredients to a blender.
- Blitz at high speed for 1 minute.
- Serve chilled.

Honey Apple cider Vinegar Drink

Ingredients

Two tablespoons honey

Two tablespoons apple cider vinegar

One glass water, hot

One green tea teabag

Directions

- Boil about 1 cup of water and place your tea bag in it for 2 minutes.
- Add the honey and vinegar.
- Stir thoroughly.
- Drink warm and enjoy.

Morning Dew

Ingredients

1 ½ cup of coconut milk

1 cup mixed berries

½ cup apple, sliced

Three tablespoons oatmeal

One teaspoon chia

One tablespoon honey

Ice cubes

Directions

- Add all the ingredients to a blender.
- Blitz at high speed for 1 minute.
- Serve chilled and enjoy.

Belly Comforter

Ingredients

Five tablespoons lemon juice

½ teaspoon turmeric

Three tablespoons aloe vera

¼ teaspoon black pepper

1 cup of water

Directions

- Add all the ingredients to a blender.
- Blend until smooth.
- Serve chilled.

Ginger Tea

Ingredients

Two tablespoons ginger, grated

½ teaspoon turmeric

¼ teaspoon black pepper

Three tablespoons lemon

One green tea teabag

1 ½ cup water

Directions

- Pour the water into a kettle and allow to boil.
- Add the ginger to the boiling water and cook for about 3 - 5 minutes.
- Take the kettle away from the heat and add the other ingredients.
- Stir well and serve warm.

Cinnamon Drink

Ingredients

Three tablespoons honey

½ teaspoon black pepper

One teaspoon ginger

One teaspoon cinnamon

2 cups of water

Directions

- Boil some water and add the ginger followed by the pepper and cinnamon.

- Allow boiling for 1 minute.
- Pour into a cup and allow to cool for about 1 minute.
- Add the honey and stir well.
- Serve warm and enjoy.

Plain Water

Ingredients

Water

Directions

Drink at least eight glasses of clean water in a day.

Other Books by the Author

The Heavenly Bowls of Buddha Goodness: Mindful Cooking Recipes for Weight Loss, Healthy Living, and Mindful Eating

These Buddha Bowl recipes are not just the trending food in town; it is what your body needs and your tongue crave for at all times. A Buddha Bowl is the agglomeration of a single bowl of delicious and healthy food ingredients. It is a dish based on a balanced combination of vegetables, grains, and proteins. These food classes are not just to be obtained from any source; they should be from organic and life-giving sources that are in peace with the environment and your body.

The term Buddha Bowl tends to elicit a picture of a vegan, which is most often the case. However, the recipes cater to the needs of non-vegan individuals too. In as a lot of us are becoming more conscious of our health and eating habits, some persons who seek enlightenment through the way of Buddha will find this book exceptional helpful in meeting their nutritional requirements.

The combination of ingredients ranging from fish, meat to vegetables and grains for the Bowls is almost infinite. This is as a result of the diverse cultures and individual preferences when it comes to how the Bowl is put together. It doesn't matter what your food orientation is, there is something for you. A Buddha

Bowl is very easy to prepare with quite a lot of the components requiring little or no cooking.

This book will guide you in making meals that are mouthwatering and at the same time healthy serving as a bonus for the minimal time you spent in preparing it. There is never a dull moment with putting together a Buddha Bowl and enjoying the meal with loved ones.

Are you ready to cleanse your body with some soul-lifting food?

Are you ready to walk away from junk and polluting foods?

Do you think it is time you begin to care for the health of your body?

Looking out for those around you who you genuinely care for?

Then it is time you get this book and lovingly put the recipes and meals together for a healthy and fun filled life.

The Cannabis Cookbook Bible 3 Books in 1: Marijuana Stoner Chef Cookbook, The Healing Path with Essential CBD oil and Hemp oil 32 Delicious Cannabis infused drinks

Considering cooking with cannabis or making use of products of marijuana must have crossed your mind a few times but getting started has been an uphill task with the legal issues surrounding the use of the product. This is not an option as the ignorance, and strict hold on the availability of this plant has been eased gradually. With the regulations appearing to come to terms with the inevitability of making mainstream cannabis use, you can fully start to enjoy the amazing benefits of cannabis and its allied products.

This book is a compilation of three books; The Healing Path with Essential CBD oil and Hemp oil; The Simple Beginners Guide to Managing Anxiety Attacks, Weight Loss, Diabetes and Holistic Healing, 32 Delicious Cannabis infused drinks; Healthy marijuana appetizers, tonics, and cocktails and Marijuana Stoner Chef Cookbook A Beginners Guide to Simple, Easy and Healthy Cannabis Recipes. These books were written to start you on the path of living a healthy life free of pain and everyday discomforts, having a delicious meal with friends and family and spicing up your day.

What other reasons do you need to buy this book?

You get a beginners idea of what cannabis is all about

How to buy high-grade marijuana.

Know the great health benefits you can get from the use of cannabis and CBD oil.

Great recipes and edibles that you can make from cannabis.

Guide on how to dose using CBD oil.

How to maximize the effects of cannabis in your cooking.

Preparing cannabis-infused smoothies, cocktails and beverages that can be made from cannabis.

This book is all you need to become comfortable and have a nice relation making use of cannabis. This is a plant that can be incorporated into your everyday meals. You will also learn how you can explore this plant and derive the very best it has got to offer.

You have waited your whole life for this very moment. Don't let his minute slip by you. Get this book now explore the colorful world of cannabis!

The Healing Path with Essential CBD oil and Hemp oil: The Simple Beginner's Guide to Managing Anxiety Attacks, Weight Loss, Diabetes and Holistic Healing

Suffering from arthritis, diabetes, severe chronic pain and a host of other debilitating ailments can limit your quality of life. The constant intake of a cocktail of medications will always leave you with horrible aftermaths that were not listed on the package of such drugs. The battering and deterioration that your internal organs undergo can only just be imagined as these medications cause more damage than good in the long run.

The wholesome nature and abundant benefits that CBD oil has cannot just be overlooked. Its uses range from managing common pains and to the more complex and debilitating conditions that ravage us in this age and time. It is used for the treatment of pains, depression, irritable bowel syndrome, epilepsy and illnesses that you can never imagine will be easily handled by this compound. CBD is wholly naturally without any hint of synthetic compounds is just what you need for that immediate relief from the condition that has been keeping you down for so long.

This book is a beginner guide on what CBD and Hemp oil are, all you need to know, some of the numerous ailments that it can be used to treat, modes of preparation, how to dose on CBD and a guide of how to shop for CBD. Also addressed in this book is the nagging issues of legal barriers that are continually being surmounted with each passing day as new information on the benefits of CBD oil comes to light.

Are you ready to know how you can use CBD oil to

Boost your immune system

Have a clearer skin

Control those pains

Increase your sexual appetite

Lighten your moods

Have a good night's rest

Improve your learning and retention abilities

And have a generally healthy and wholesome lifestyle?

In this beginner's guide, you will be made aware of how CBD oil can be the best thing that ever happened to you.

So for how long are you going to cope with that pain, the condition that keeps you down most of the day? Take that all critical, decisive step now, dump the medications that are not doing you any good and embrace the natural path to healing.

Get this book now!

Cannabis Bud Smoothie: Healthy Medicinal Drinks and Marijuana Infusions

Quite a lot of folks with chronic medical conditions are sceptical about the consumption of marijuana by smoking it. If you are in this category, then here is an easy way out. Taking in medicinal cannabis by adding it to your delicious smoothies and juicing it will give you all the health benefits and much more! Ingesting of cannabis fresh and raw is the most advantageous as all the nutrients, and cannabinoid compounds will remain intact without undergoing any change into compounds that you may not necessarily need at this point.

You will learn how to incorporate cannabis buds and cannabis infusions into your daily smoothies to aid you in managing those severe pains, inflammations, ailments and generally giving you a more healthy life.

This book is filled with a delicious smoothie, and juice recipes packed loaded with vitamins, nutrients and cannabinoids. The recipes are organic, gluten and sugar-free with the foundation been cannabis.

In this book, you will learn;

The great health benefits of cannabis

How to prepare delicious smoothies and juices

Ease away those excruciating pains

And so much more!

BUY this book today and begin your journey towards a more healthier life!

Cannabis Cultivation and Horticulture: The Simple Guide to Growing Marijuana Indoors Using Hydroponics

This is an excellent guide for beginners and professionals alike on the indoor cultivation of marijuana for personal use using hydroponics and soil. It brings to you the simple techniques and methods need to have a thriving sanctuary for your cannabis plants and produce plants with potent buds and massive amounts of resins! Cultivating your cannabis indoors gives you the opportunity to monitor its growth and make adjustments to the environmental conditions that will significantly stimulate the growth of the plant. It is also an avenue to prevent the pestilence that comes with outdoor cultivation. Looking to have a basic knowledge that can be leveraged to grow great plants? Then this is the book for you!

Major and minor parts involved in the cultivation of cannabis are thoroughly handled. From the design and type of sanctuary space to the kind of nutrients, lightning to temperature, pest control to flow of air; everything you need to grow potent strains of marijuana is just within your grasp. Each stage of cultivation from obtaining the seeds to drying and curing is fully explained in terms that you can easily understand and put to practice immediately.

So do you want to take the first steps towards nurturing this beautiful plant from seed to a potent wonder of nature? This book will teach you how to

Grow your stash while employing high safety standards

Learn how to secure a discrete growing space in a confined area

Have the ability to determine the potency of your product

Force flowering

Applying the best nutrients formulas to your plants

Crossing and identifying the best strain for you

Getting all unfertilized female plants (Sensimilla)

Controlling Pests

Making the best use of the hydroponics

And so much more!

Getting started with this book will make you an enlightened cultivator and appreciator of everything cannabis and not just a grower. BUY this book now and have a high time!

About the Author

Rina S. Gritton has been all about healthy intake of food and living the life of a real food aficionado. With her it is about food, making us of spices, herbs, and other ingredients around in nature that ensures we all stay at the peak of our health at all times.

She has been putting together great recipes and meals as a hobby and business to loved ones and clients alike. What started as a challenge to help her parents and siblings

eat better turned to a full-fledged campaign and career in making use of purely organic foods and materials around us.

A dietician with several years experience in the treatment of dietary issues and business owner catering for the desires of folks to have organic and tasteful meals, she also guest writes for blogs, websites, and volunteers in cooking classes in high schools.

She lives in Santa Monica, California with her husband and children.

Printed in Great Britain
by Amazon